My Mediterranean Diet Plan

*Easy, fast
and low-calorie recipes
for a healthy lifestyle
and weight loss*

Carlo Montesanti

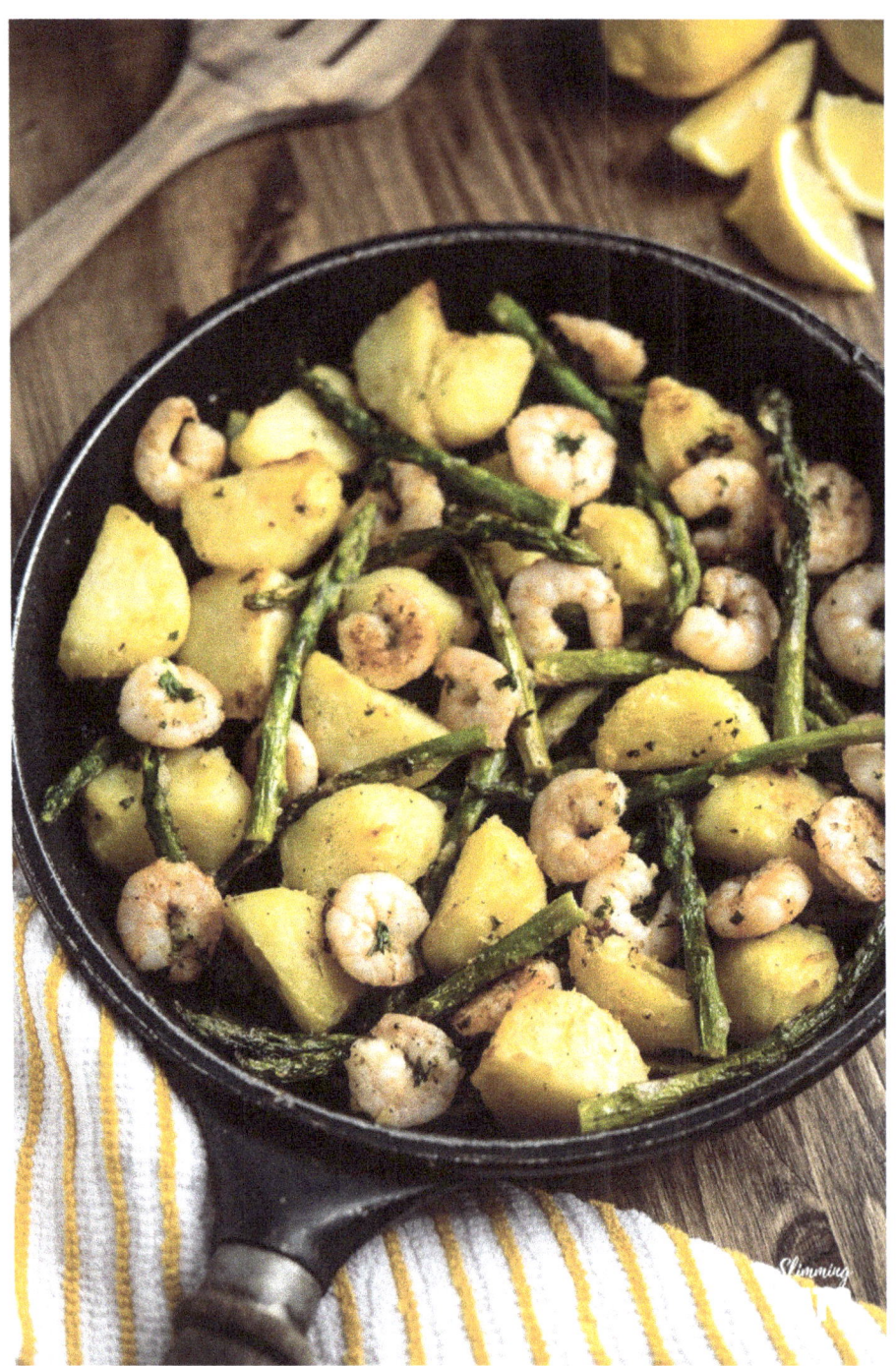

© copyright 2021 – all rights reserved.

the content contained within this book may not be reproduced, duplicated or transmitted without direct written permission from the author or the publisher.

under no circumstances will any blame or legal responsibility be held against the publisher, or author, for any damages, reparation, or monetary loss due to the information contained within this book. either directly or indirectly.

legal notice:

this book is copyright protected. this book is only for personal use. you cannot amend, distribute, sell, use, quote or paraphrase any part, or the content within this book, without the consent of the author or publisher.

disclaimer notice:

please note the information contained within this document is for educational and entertainment purposes only. all effort has been executed to present accurate, up to date, and reliable, complete information. no warranties of any kind are declared or implied. readers acknowledge that the author is not engaging in the rendering of legal, financial, medical or professional advice. the content within this book has been derived from various sources. please consult a licensed professional before attempting any techniques outlined in this book.

by reading this document, the reader agrees that under no circumstances is the author responsible for any losses, direct or indirect, which are incurred as a result of the use of information contained within this document, including, but not limited to, — errors, omissions, or inaccuracies.

Table of Contents

- Braised Leek with Pine Nuts 6
- Parsley Butter Shrimp 8
- Foil Baked Salmon 10
- Baked Zesty Tilapia 12
- Prawns with Asparagus 15
- Tuna and Kale 17
- Minty Soup 19
- Special Orzo Soup 21
- Sweet and gorgeous Lentil Stew 23
- Delicious Meatball Soup for the Spanish 25
- Rice Rolls 27
- Rice Stew with Squid 29
- Creamy Millet 31
- Oatmeal Cakes 32
- Yogurt Buckwheat 34
- Halloumi Buckwheat Bowl 35
- Aromatic Green Millet 37
- Quinoa with Pumpkin 38
- Almond Quinoa 39
- Spring Rolls with Quinoa 42
- Mushroom Quinoa Skillet 44
- Strawberry Quinoa Bowl 46
- Quinoa Meatballs 48
- Stir-Fried Farro 50
- Quick Farro Skillet 51
- Bulgur Bowl 53
- Boiled Bulgur with Kale 54
- Chicken and Rice Soup 55
- Tomato Bulgur 57
- Well spiced Lentil Soup with sour taste 58

- Delicious and entertaining Lamb Veggie Soup 60
- Aromatic Baked Brown Rice 62
- Aromatic Barley Pilaf 65
- Basmati Rice Pilaf Mix 67
- Brown Rice Salad with Asparagus, Goat Cheese, and Lemon 69
- Carrot-Almond-Bulgur Salad 73
- Chickpea-Spinach Bulgur 75
- Classic Baked Brown Rice 77
- Classic Italian Seafood Risotto 79
- Classic Stovetop White Rice 83
- Chicken Sausage Minestrone 85
- Italian Lentil soup 88
- Smoked chicken sausage soup 90
- Bulgur, Kale and Cheese Mix 92
- Lemon Chicken Soup 94
- Tuscan Vegetable Pasta Soup 96
- Dairy Free Zucchini Soup 99
- Farro Stew with Kale & Cannellini Beans 101
- Italian Meatball Soup 104

Braised Leek with Pine Nuts

Prep Time: 45 min

Cook Time: 15 min

Serve: 2

Ingredients:

- tbsp. Ghee
- tsp Olive oil pieces Leek
- oz. Vegetable broth
- A bunch of fresh parsley
- 1 tbsp. fresh oregano
- 1 tbsp. Pine nuts (roasted)

Preparation:

1. Cut the leek into thin rings and finely chop the herbs. Roast the pine nuts in a dry pan over medium heat.

2. Melt the ghee together with the olive oil in a large pan. Cook the leek until golden brown for 5 minutes, stirring constantly.

3. Add the vegetable broth and cook for another 10 minutes until the leek is tender. Stir in the herbs and sprinkle the pine nuts on the dish just before serving.

Parsley Butter Shrimp

Prep Time: 10 min

Cook Time: 22 min

Serve: 4

Ingredients:

- 1 lb. shrimp, peeled and deveined
- tbsp. butter, divided
- cloves garlic, minced
- ½ cup chicken stock
- tbsp. parsley, minced
- tbsp. Lemon juice
- ¼ tsp. Red pepper flakes
- ½ tsp. Black pepper
- ½ tsp. kosher salt

Preparation:

1. Heat 2 tbsp. of butter in a large, heavy-bottomed skillet over medium heat. Add the shrimp to the skillet and sprinkle with salt and pepper.

2. Cook, occasionally stirring, for 5 minutes or until shrimp is cooked through. Remove shrimp to a plate and set aside.

3. Add the garlic to the skillet and cook, constantly stirring, for 30 seconds. Add the chicken stock and whisk to combine. Simmer until the stock has reduced by half, about 7 minutes.

4. Add the remaining 4 tbsp. of butter, lemon juice, and red pepper to the sauce. Stir to melt the butter and cook for two more minutes.

5. Remove from heat and return the shrimp to the sauce. Sprinkle the parsley over the top and stir to combine. Serve immediately.

Foil Baked Salmon

Prep Time: 8 min

Cook Time: 20 min

Serve: 2

Ingredients:

- salmon fillets
- asparagus spears
- 1 tsp. dried oregano
- slices onion
- 1 tsp. fresh parsley, chopped
- slices lemon
- 1 tbsp. extra virgin olive oil
- Salt and black pepper to taste

Preparation:

1. Preheat oven to 400° F. In a medium bowl, place the two pieces of salmon. Pour 1 tbsp. Of olive oil and sprinkle salt, pepper, and dried oregano.

2. Cut two sheets of foil. It has to be big enough to wrap the salmon and asparagus. First place asparagus, about 8 spears, on the sheet of foil. Layer fillets over asparagus, then top each with about two onion slices and two lemon slices.

3. Wrap sides of foil inward over salmon, fold on top and bottom of the foil to enclose. Place foil packets in a single layer on a baking sheet.

4. Bake in preheated oven for about 15 minutes. Unwrap and using a large spatula, transfer the foil packets to plates. Serve warm!

Baked Zesty Tilapia

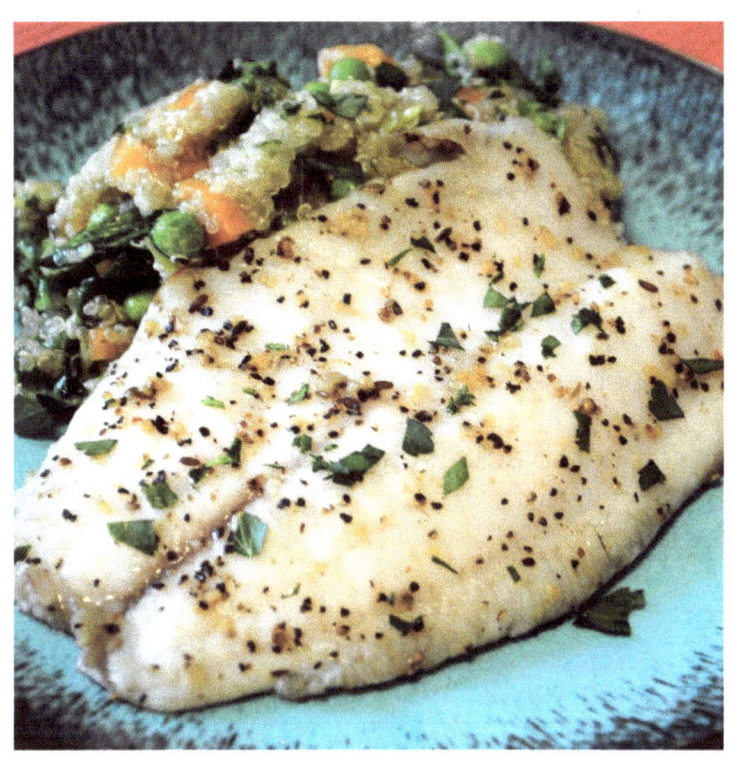

Prep Time: 10 min

Cook Time: 10 min

Serve: 4

Ingredients:

- tilapia fillets
- ¼ cup unsalted butter, melted cloves
- garlic, minced
- tbsp. freshly squeezed lemon juice to taste
- Zest of 1 lemon
- tbsp. chopped fresh parsley leaves
- Kosher salt and black pepper to taste

Preparation:

1. Preheat the oven to 425° F. Lightly grease a baking dish or coat with non-stick spray. In a small bowl, whisk together butter, lemon juice, garlic, and lemon zest and set aside.

2. Season the fillets with salt and pepper, taste and place onto the prepared baking dish and drizzle with butter mixture.

3. Place into the oven and bake until fish flakes easily with a fork, about 10 minutes. Serve immediately, garnished with parsley.

Prawns with Asparagus

Prep Time: 10 min

Cook Time: 12 min

Serve: 4

Ingredients:

- tbsp. olive oil
- 1 lb. prawns, peeled, and deveined
- 1 lb. asparagus, trimmed
- Salt and black pepper, to taste
- 1 tsp. garlic, minced
- 1 tsp. fresh ginger, minced
- 1 tbsp. low-sodium soy sauce
- tbsp. lemon juice

Preparation:

1. In a wok, heat 2 tbsp. of oil over medium-high heat and cook the prawns with salt and black pepper for

about 4 minutes. With a slotted spoon, transfer the prawns into a bowl and set aside.

2. In the same wok, heat remaining 1 tbsp. Of oil over medium-high heat and cook the asparagus, ginger, garlic, salt, and black pepper and sauté for about 7 minutes, stirring frequently. Stir in the prawns and soy sauce and cook for about 1 minute.

3. Stir in the lemon juice and remove from the heat. Serve hot.

Tuna and Kale

Prep Time: 5 min

Cook Time: 20 min

Serve: 4

Ingredients:

- 1 lb. tuna fillets, boneless, skinless and cubed
- tbsp. olive oil
- 1 cup kale, torn
- ½ cup cherry tomatoes, cubed
- 1 yellow onion, chopped

Preparation:

1. Heat a pan with the oil over medium heat. Add the onion and sauté for 5 minutes. Add the tuna and the other ingredients.

2. Toss and cook everything for 15 minutes more, divide between plates and serve.

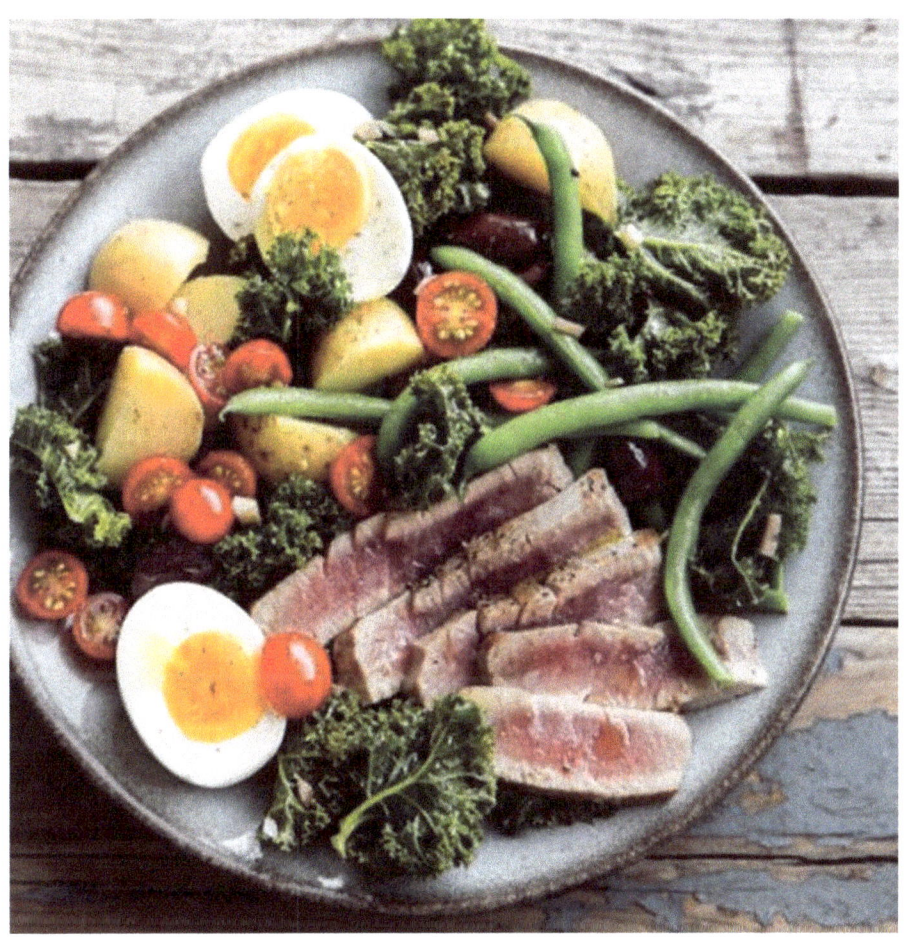

Minty Soup

Prep and Cook Time: 35 min

Serve: 6

Ingredients:

- chopped garlic cloves – 2
- water – 1 cup
- olive oil – 2 tbsps
- heavy cream – ¼ cup
- vegetable stock – 2 cups
- chopped shallots - 2
- lemon juice – 1 tbsp
- chopped mint leaves - 4
- dried oregano – ½ tsp
- Pepper and salt to taste
- pound green peas - 1

Preparation:

1. In garlic and shallots, stir heated oil in a soup pot and cook until it's softened for 2 minutes. Then add oregano, green peas, stock, mint and water.

2. Cook for 15 minutes on a low heat after adding pepper and salt to taste. In the lemon juice, stir and cook it for 2 more minutes.

3. Remove from heat when it is done and stir it in the cream. Use an immersion blender to puree the soup immersion blender until it is smooth and creamy. Best served chilled or warm.

Special Orzo Soup

Cook and Prep Time: 45 min

Serve: 8

Ingredients:

- Orzo – ¼ cup
- vegetable stock – 2 cups
- lemon juice – 2 tbsps
- cored and diced yellow bell pepper - 1
- extra virgin olive oil – 2 tbsps
- chopped shallots - 2
- baby spinach – 4 cups
- green peas – 1 cup
- cored and diced green bell pepper - 1
- water – 4 cups
- chopped garlic cloves - 2
- Pepper and salt to taste

Preparation:

1. In a soup pot, heat the oil and stir in the garlic and shallots. Add other Ingredients: after cooking it for 2 minutes and season with pepper and salt.

2. On low heat, cook it for 25 minutes. Best served chilled or warm.

Sweet and gorgeous Lentil Stew

Cook and Prep Time: 45 min

Serve: 8

Ingredients:

- water – 3 cups
- crushed tomatoes – 1 can
- extra virgin olive oil – 2 tbsps
- chopped garlic cloves – 2
- diced carrots - 2
- cored and diced red bell peppers - 2
- diced celery stalk – 1
- cumin seeds – ½ tsp
- mustard seeds – ½ tsp
- chopped shallots - 2
- vegetable stock – 3 cups

- Pepper and salt to taste
- green lentils – 1 cup
- Yogurt for serving

Preparation:

1. In a soup pot, heat the oil and stir in the garlic and shallots. Add other Ingredients: after cooking it for 2 minutes. On low heat, adjust the taste with pepper and salt for 30 minutes.

2. Top it with freshly chopped parsley or plain yogurt after serving the soup fresh and warm.

Delicious Meatball Soup for the Spanish

Cook and Prep Time: 1 h

Serve: 8

Ingredients:

- water – 6 cups
- crushed tomatoes – 1 can
- egg - 1
- olive oil – 2 tbsps
- diced celery stalk - 1
- chopped onion - 1
- cored and diced red bell peppers – 2
- vegetable stock – 2 cups
- diced carrots - 2
- pound ground veal - 1
- chopped parsley – 2 tbsps

- chopped garlic cloves - 2
- Pepper and salt to taste

Preparation:

1. In a soup pot, heat the oil and stir in the garlic, stock, bell peppers, onions, carrots, water and celery. Bring to a boiling after seasoning with pepper and salt.

2. In a bowl, mix egg, veal and parsley in the meantime. Then boil them in boiling liquid after forming small meatballs. Adjust the taste with pepper and salt after adding the tomatoes. For 20 minutes, cook on very low heat. Best served fresh and warm.

Rice Rolls

Prep Time: 15 min

Cook Time: 35 min

Serve: 6

Ingredients:

- 4 white cabbage leaves
- 4 oz ground chicken
- ½ tsp. garlic powder
- ¼ cup of long grain rice, cooked
- ½ cup chicken stock
- ½ cup tomatoes, chopped

Preparation:

1. In the bowl, mix ground chicken, garlic powder, and rice.

2. Then put the rice mixture on every cabbage leaf and roll.

3. Arrange the rice rolls in the saucepan. Add chicken stock and tomatoes and close the lid.

4. Cook the rice rolls for 35 minutes on low heat.

Rice Stew with Squid

Prep Time: 10 min

Cook Time: 30 min

Serve: 6

Ingredients:

- 5 oz long grain rice
- 4 oz squid, sliced
- 1 jalapeno pepper, chopped
- ½ cup tomatoes, chopped
- 1 onion, diced
- 2 cups chicken stock
- 1 tbsp. avocado oil

Preparation:

1. Roast the onion with avocado oil in the skillet for 3-4 minutes or until the onion is light brown. Add squid, jalapeno pepper, and tomatoes. Cook the ingredients for 7 minutes. Then cook rice with water for 15 minutes.

2. Add cooked rice in the squid mixture, stir, and cook for 3 minutes more.

Creamy Millet

Prep Time: 10 min

Cook Time: 10 min

Serve: 6

Ingredients:

- ½ cup millet
- 1 oz cream cheese
- ¼ tsp. salt
- 1.5 cup hot water

Preparation:

Mix hot water and millet in the saucepan. Boil it for 8 minutes on low heat. Add cream cheese and salt. Carefully stir the cooked millet.

Oatmeal Cakes

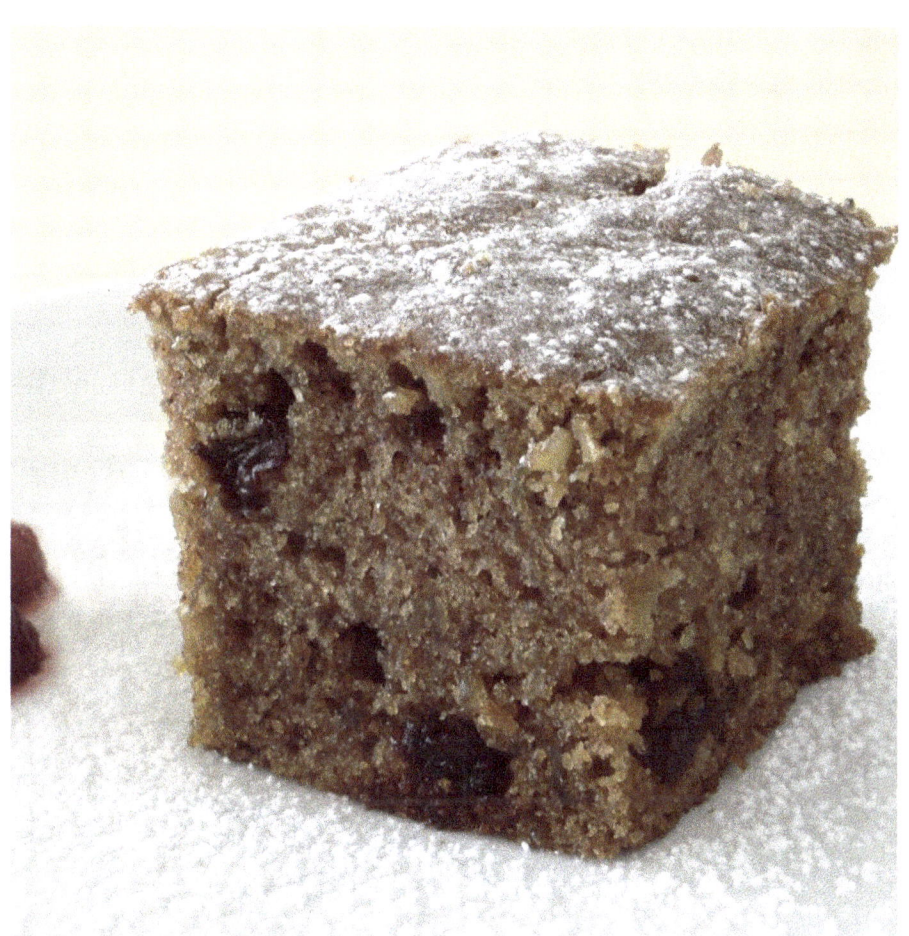

Prep Time: 15 min

Cook Time: 7 min

Serve: 4

Ingredients:

- ½ cup oatmeal

- 1 egg, beaten
- 1 carrot, grated
- 1 tbsp. olive oil
- 1 tsp. flax meal
-

Preparation

1. Put oatmeal, egg, grated carrot, and flax meal in the blender. Blend the mixture well. Then heat olive oil in the skillet.

2. Make the medium-sized cakes from the oatmeal mixture and cook for 3 minutes per side on medium heat.

Yogurt Buckwheat

Prep Time: 5 min

Cook Time: 13 min

Serve: 2

Ingredients:

- ½ cup buckwheat
- 1.5 cup chicken stock
- 1 tbsp. plain yogurt

Preparation:

Put all ingredients in the saucepan and close the lid. Cook the meal for 13 minutes on low heat or until the buckwheat soaks all liquid. Carefully stir the cooked meal.

Halloumi Buckwheat Bowl

Prep Time: 10 min

Cook Time: 15 min

Serve: 4

Ingredients:

- 1 cup buckwheat
- cups chicken stock
- 4 oz halloumi cheese
- 1 tbsp. olive oil
- ½ tsp. dried thyme

Preparation:

1. Mix chicken stock and buckwheat in the saucepan, boil, and cook for 7 minutes on medium heat. After this, sprinkle the halloumi cheese with olive oil and dried thyme.

2. Grill it for 2 minutes per side or until the cheese is light brown. Then put the cooked buckwheat in the bowls.

3. Chop the cheese roughly and top the buckwheat with it.

Aromatic Green Millet

Prep Time: 10 min

Cook Time: 7 min

Serve: 5

Ingredients:

- 1 cup millet
- 2 cups of water
- 4 tbsp. pesto sauce
- ¼ tsp. cayenne pepper
-
- **Preparation:**

1. Mix water and millet in the saucepan and boil for 7 minutes. Then add cayenne pepper and pesto sauce.

2. Stir the millet until homogenous and green.

Quinoa with Pumpkin

Prep Time: 5 min

Cook Time: 20 min

Serve: 6

Ingredients:

- ½ cup pumpkin, cubed
- 1 tbsp. lemon juice
- 1 tsp. liquid honey
- 1 cup quinoa
- 2 cups of water
- ¼ cup of organic almond milk

Preparation:

1. Put almond milk and pumpkin in the saucepan. Add lemon juice and water. Cook the pumpkin for 10 minutes.

2. Then add quinoa and cook the meal for 10 minutes.

3. Remove the cooked meal from the heat, add liquid honey, and stir well.

Almond Quinoa

Prep Time: 5 min

Cook Time: 4 min

Serve: 4

Ingredients:

- 1 cup quinoa
- 2 cups of water
- 1 cup organic almond milk
- ½ cup strawberries, sliced
- 1 tbsp. honey

Preparation:

1. Pour water and milk in the saucepan and bring to boil.

2. Add quinoa and cook it for 12 minutes. Then cool the cooked quinoa and add honey. Stir.

3. Transfer the quinoa in the bowls and top with strawberries.

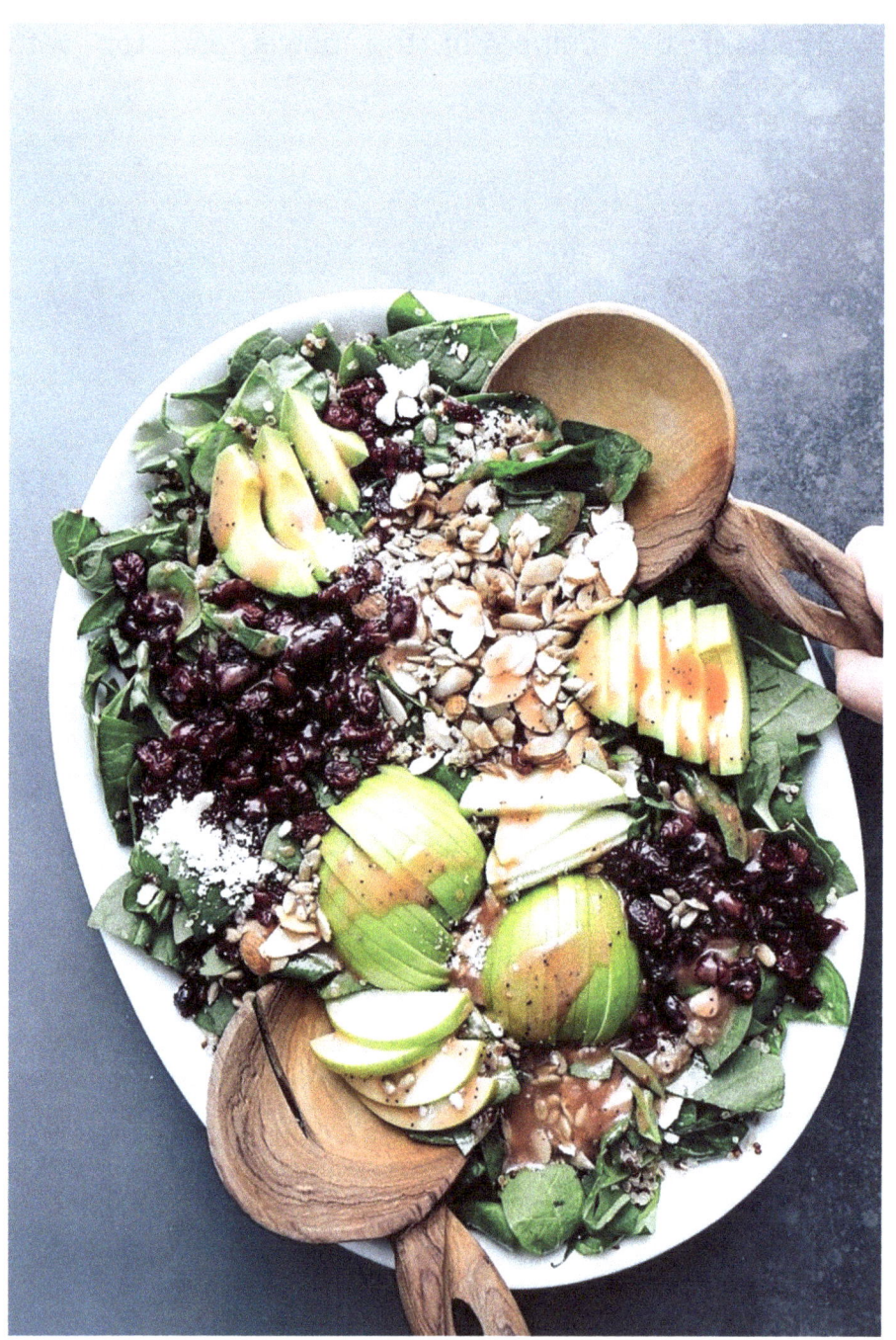

Spring Rolls with Quinoa

Prep Time: 10 min

Cook Time: 1 min

Serve: 8

Ingredients:

- 8 rice pepper wraps
- 1 cup quinoa, cooked
- 1 carrot, cut into strips
- 1 cup lettuce leaves
- 1 tbsp. olive oil

Preparation:

1. Make the rice pepper wraps wet. Then put the cooked quinoa on every rice pepper wrap.

2. Add carrot and lettuce leaves and wrap them into the rolls. Brush every roll with olive oil and put it in the hot skillet. Roast the spring rolls for 20 seconds per side.

Mushroom Quinoa Skillet

Prep Time: 10 min

Cook Time: 25 min

Serve: 6

Ingredients:

- 1 cup mushrooms, sliced
- ½ cup of water
- 1 tbsp. olive oil
- 1 tsp. Italian seasonings
- ½ cup quinoa
- ½ cup organic almond milk
- ¼ tsp. dried thyme

Preparation:

1. Roast mushrooms with olive oil in the saucepan for 10 minutes. Then stir them well, add Italian seasonings, dried thyme, and quinoa.

2. Add almond milk and water.

3. Close the lid and simmer the meal for 15 minutes. Stir it from time to time to avoid burning.

Strawberry Quinoa Bowl

Prep Time: 15 min

Cook Time: 0 min

Serve: 8

Ingredients:

- 2 ½ cup quinoa, cooked
- ¼ cup strawberries, roughly chopped
- ½ cup fresh spinach, chopped
- 2 pecans, chopped
- 1 tbsp. balsamic vinegar
- 1 tsp. avocado oil

Preparation:

1. Mix quinoa, fresh spinach, and pecans in the big bowl.

2. Then add strawberries and avocado oil. Gently shake the mixture and transfer in the serving bowls.

3. Sprinkle every serving with a small amount of balsamic vinegar.

Quinoa Meatballs

Prep Time: 15 min

Cook Time: 30 min

Serve: 6

Ingredients:

- ½ cup quinoa, cooked
- ½ cup ground pork
- 1 tbsp. chives, chopped
- 1 egg, beaten
- 1 tbsp. sesame seeds
- 1 tsp. chili flakes
- 1 cup tomato juice

Preparation:

1. In the bowl mi quinoa, ground pork, chives, egg, sesame seeds, and chili flakes. Then make the small meatballs and put them in the baking pan.

2. Top the meatballs with tomato juice and cook in the preheated to 375F oven for 30 minutes.

Stir-Fried Farro

Prep Time: 10 min

Cook Time: 8 min

Serve: 4

Ingredients:

- 1 cup farro, cooked
- 1 egg, beaten
- 1 tbsp. olive oil
- ½ tsp. chili flakes

Preparation:

1. Heat olive oil and egg beaten egg. Cook it for 1 minute and then stir it carefully. Add cooked farro and chili flakes.

2. Fry the meal for 7 minutes. Stir it from time to time.

Quick Farro Skillet

Prep Time: 10 min

Cook Time: 15 min

Serve: 6

Ingredients:

- 2 oz fresh spinach, chopped
- 2 oz asparagus, chopped
- 1/3 cup farro, cooked
- 1 tbsp. olive oil
- ½ tsp. curry powder

Preparation:

Line the skillet with baking paper. Put all ingredients in the prepared skillet, flatten them gently and transfer in the preheated to 365°F oven. Cook the meal for 15 minutes.

Bulgur Bowl

Prep Time: 10 min

Cook Time: 0 min

Serve: 4

Ingredients:

- 6 oz salmon, boiled, chopped
- ½ cup bulgur, cooked
- 1 cup fresh cilantro, chopped
- 1 cup tomato, chopped
- 3 tbsp. lemon juice
- 1 tbsp. olive oil

Preparation:

Put salmon, bulgur, cilantro, and tomato in the bowl. Add lemon juice and olive oil. Shake the mixture well and transfer in the serving bowls.

Boiled Bulgur with Kale

Prep Time: 10 min

Cook Time: 11 min

Serve: 6

Ingredients:

- 1 cup bulgur cups water
- 1 cup kale
- ½ zucchini, chopped
- ½ tsp. allspices
- 6 tbsp. olive oil
- 2 oz goat cheese, crumbled

Preparation:

1. Mix water and bulgur in the saucepan and cook boil for 11 minutes. Then cool the bulgur and mix it with chopped kale, zucchini, allspices, and olive oil.

2. Transfer the bulgur meal in the serving bowls and top with goat cheese.

Chicken and Rice Soup

Prep Time: 10 min

Cook Time: 20 min

Serve: 6

Ingredients:

- 4 cups chicken stock
- 1 cup of water
- 1-lb. chicken breast, shredded
- 1 cup of rice, cooked
- 3 egg yolks
- 3 tbsp. lemon juice
- 1/3 cup fresh parsley, chopped
- ½ tsp. salt
- ¼ tsp. ground black pepper

Preparation:

1. Pour water and chicken stock in the saucepan and bring to boil. Then pour one cup of the hot liquid in the food processor.

2. Add cooked rice, egg yolks, lemon juice, and salt. Blend the mixture until smooth. After this, transfer the smooth rice mixture into the saucepan with remaining chicken stock liquid.

3. Add shredded chicken breast, parsley, and ground black pepper. Boil the soup for 5 minutes more.

Tomato Bulgur

Prep Time: 5 min

Cook Time: 20 min

Serve: 3

Ingredients:

- ½ cup bulgur
- 1 onion, diced
- 3 tbsp. tomato paste
- ½ tsp. salt
- 2 tbsp. olive oil
- 1 cup of water

Preparation:

Melt the olive oil in the saucepan. Add diced onion and cook it until light brown. Then add bulgur and tomato paste. Stir the ingredients. Add water and cook the meal for 15 minutes.

Well spiced Lentil Soup with sour taste

Cook and Prep Time: 45 min

Serve: 6

Ingredients:

- water – 6 cups
- diced celery stalk - 1
- olive oil – 2 tbsps
- oregano sprig - 1
- chopped shallot – 1
- thyme sprig - 1
- chopped garlic clove – 1
- diced tomatoes – ½ cup
- cored and diced green bell pepper – 1
- sliced rhubarb stalks - 4
- cored and diced yellow bell pepper – 1

- green lentils – 1 cup
- diced carrot - 1
- vegetable stock – 2 cups
- Salt and pepper to taste

Preparation:

1. In a soup pot, heat the oil and stir in the garlic, bell peppers, shallots, carrot and celery. Soften it by cooking for 5 minutes and add stock, the lentils, water, rhubarb and water, also add tomatoes.

2. Add oregano sprig and thyme after seasoning with pepper and salt. For 20 minutes, cook on low heat. Best served chilled or warm.

Delicious and entertaining Lamb Veggie Soup

Cook and Prep Time: 1 ½ h

Serve: 8

Ingredients:

- water – 6 cups
- cubed pound lamb shoulder – 1 1 2
- lemon juice – 2 tbsps
- cauliflower florets – 2 cups
- olive oil – 2 tbsps
- basil sprig - 1
- chopped shallots – 2
- crushed tomatoes – 1 can
- diced carrots – 2

- thyme sprig - 1
- diced celery stalks – 2
- green peas – ½ cup
- grated ginger – ¼ tsp
- vegetable stock – 4 cups
- oregano sprig - 1
- Pepper and salt to taste
-

Preparation:

1. In a soup pot, heat the oil and stir in the lamb shoulder. Add stock and water after cooking on all sides for 5 minutes.

2. Add the remaining Ingredients: after cooking for 40 minutes and season with pepper and salt.

3. Cook it for another 20 minutes and serve the soup when it's still fresh.

Aromatic Baked Brown Rice

Prep Time: 10 min

Cook Time: 20 min

Serve: 6

Ingredients:

- ½ cup minced fresh parsley
- ¾ cup jarred roasted
- red peppers, rinsed, patted dry, and chopped
- 1 cup chicken or vegetable broth
- 1½ cups long-grain brown rice, rinsed
- 2 onions, chopped fine
- 2¼ cups water
- 4 tsp. extra-virgin olive oil
- Grated Parmesan cheese
- Lemon wedges
- Salt and pepper

Preparation:

1. Place the oven rack in the centre of the oven and pre-heat your oven to 375°F. Heat oil in a Dutch oven on moderate heat until it starts to shimmer. Put in onions and 1 tsp. salt and cook, stirring intermittently, till they become tender and well browned, 12 to 14 minutes.

2. Mix in water and broth and bring to boil. Mix in rice, cover, and move pot to oven. Bake until rice becomes soft and liquid is absorbed, 65 to 70 minutes.

3. Remove pot from oven. Sprinkle red peppers over rice, cover, and allow to sit for about five minutes. Put in parsley to rice and fluff gently with fork to combine. Sprinkle with salt and pepper to taste. Serve with grated Parmesan and lemon wedges.

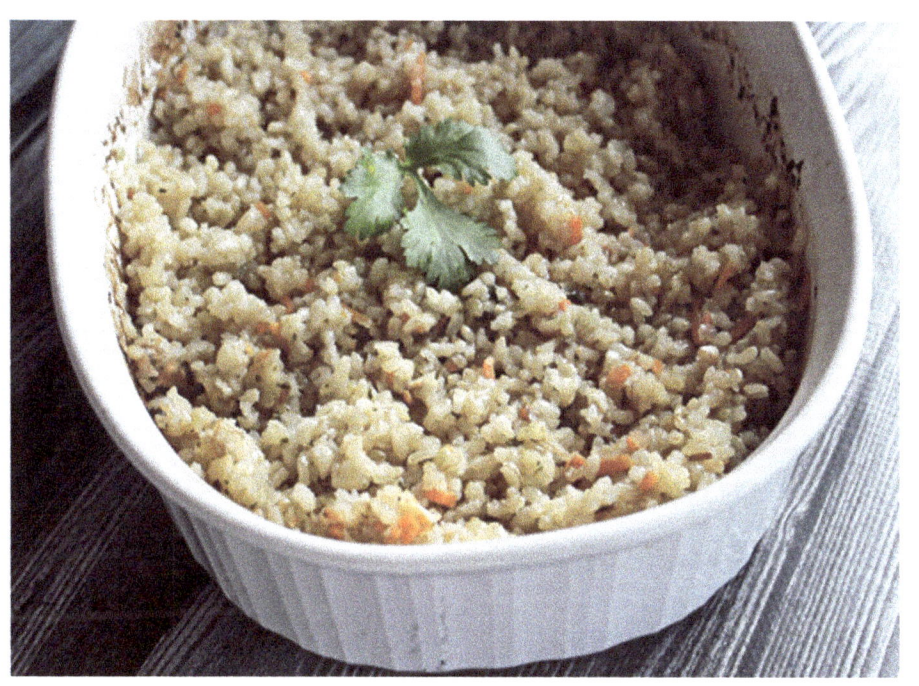

Aromatic Barley Pilaf

Prep Time: 10 min

Cook Time: 10 min

Serve: 6

Ingredients:

- ¼ cup minced fresh parsley
- 1 small onion, chopped fine
- 1½ cups pearl barley, rinsed
- 1½ tsp. lemon juice
- 1½ tsp. minced fresh thyme or ½ tsp. dried
- 2 garlic cloves, minced
- 2 tbsp. minced fresh chives
- 2½ cups water
- 3 tbsp. extra-virgin olive oil
- Salt and pepper

Preparation:

1. Heat oil in a big saucepan on moderate heat until it starts to shimmer. Put in onion and ½ tsp. salt and cook till they become tender, approximately five minutes. Mix in barley, garlic, and thyme and cook, stirring often, until barley is lightly toasted and aromatic, approximately three minutes.

2. Mix in water and bring to simmer. Decrease heat to low, cover, and simmer until barley becomes soft and water is absorbed, 20 to 40 minutes.

3. Remove from the heat, lay clean dish towel underneath lid and let pilaf sit for about ten minutes. Put in parsley, chives, and lemon juice to pilaf and fluff gently with fork to combine. Sprinkle with salt and pepper to taste. Serve.

Basmati Rice Pilaf Mix

Prep Time: 10 min

Cook Time: 15 min

Ingredients:

- ¼ cup currants
- ¼ cup sliced almonds, toasted
- ¼ tsp. ground cinnamon
- ½ tsp. ground turmeric
- 1 small onion, chopped fine
- 1 tbsp. extra-virgin olive oil
- 1½ cups basmati rice, rinsed
- 2 garlic cloves, minced
- 2¼ cups water
- Salt and pepper

Preparation:

1. Heat oil in a big saucepan on moderate heat until it starts to shimmer. Put in onion and ¼ tsp. salt and cook till they become tender, approximately five minutes. Put in rice, garlic, turmeric, and cinnamon and cook, stirring often, until grain edges begin to turn translucent, approximately three minutes.

2. Mix in water and bring to simmer. Decrease heat to low, cover, and simmer gently until rice becomes soft and water is absorbed, 16 to 18 minutes.

3. Remove from the heat, drizzle currants over pilaf. Cover, laying clean dish towel underneath lid, and let pilaf sit for about ten minutes. Put in almonds to pilaf and fluff gently with fork to combine. Sprinkle with salt and pepper to taste.

Brown Rice Salad with Asparagus, Goat Cheese, and Lemon

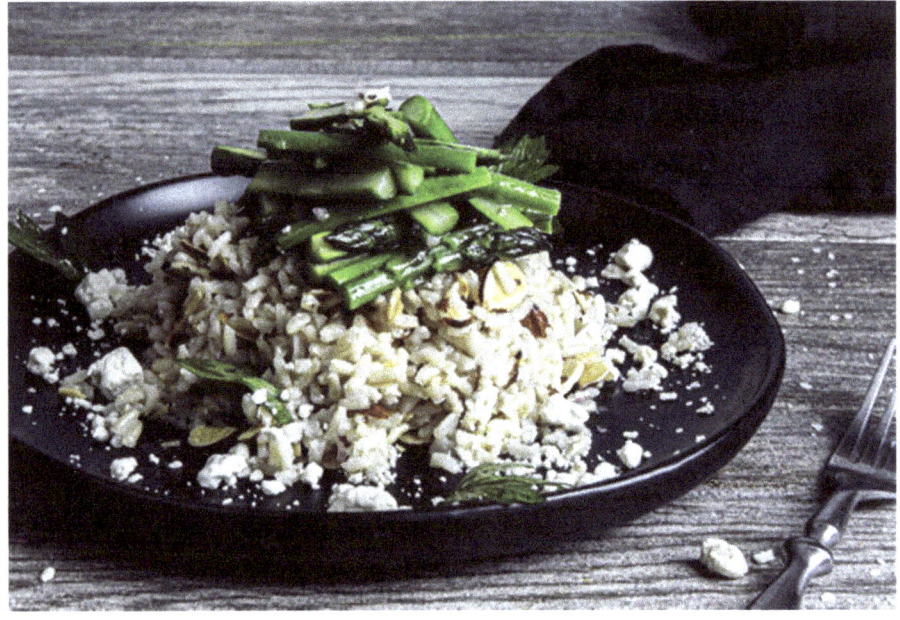

Prep Time: 10 min

Cook Time: 15 min

Serve: 2

Ingredients:

- ¼ cup minced fresh parsley
- ¼ cup slivered almonds, toasted
- 1 lb. asparagus, trimmed and cut into 1-inch lengths 1 shallot, minced
- 1 tsp. grated lemon zest plus
- 3 tbsp. juice
- 1½ cups long-grain brown rice
- 2 oz. goat cheese, crumbled (½ cup)
- 3½ tbsp. extra-virgin olive oil
- Salt and pepper

Preparation:

1. Bring 4 quarts water to boil in a Dutch oven. Put in rice and 1½ tsp. salt and cook, stirring intermittently, until rice is tender, about half an hour. Drain rice, spread onto rimmed baking sheet, and drizzle with 1 tbsp. lemon juice. Allow it to cool completely, about fifteen minutes.

2. Heat 1 tbsp. oil in 12-inch frying pan on high heat until just smoking. Put in asparagus, ¼ tsp. salt, and ¼ tsp. pepper and cook, stirring intermittently, until asparagus is browned and crisp-tender, about 4 minutes; move to plate and allow to cool slightly.

3. Beat remaining 2½ tbsp. oil, lemon zest and remaining 2 tbsp. juice, shallot, ½ tsp. salt, and ½ tsp. pepper together in a big container. Put in rice, asparagus, 2 tbsp. goat cheese, 3 tbsp. almonds, and 3 tbsp. parsley. Gently toss to combine and allow to sit

for about ten minutes. Sprinkle with salt and pepper to taste.

4. Move to serving platter and drizzle with remaining 2 tbsp. goat cheese, remaining 1 tbsp. almonds, and remaining 1 tbsp. parsley. Serve.

Carrot-Almond-Bulgur Salad

Prep Time: 10 min

Cook Time: 20 min

Serve: 4

Ingredients:

- 1/8 tsp. cayenne pepper
- 1/3 cup chopped fresh cilantro
- 1/3 cup chopped fresh mint
- 1/3 cup extra-virgin olive oil
- ½ cup sliced almonds, toasted
- ½ tsp. ground cumin
- 1 cup water
- 1½ cups medium-grind bulgur, rinsed
- 3 scallions, sliced thin
- 4 carrots, peeled and shredded
- 6 tbsp. lemon juice (2 lemons)
- Salt and pepper

Preparation:

1. Mix bulgur, water, ¼ cup lemon juice, and ¼ tsp. salt in a container. Cover and sit at room temperature until grains are softened and liquid is fully absorbed, about 1½ hours.

2. Beat remaining 2 tbsp. lemon juice, oil, cumin, cayenne, and ½ tsp. salt together in a big container.

3. Put in bulgur, carrots, scallions, almonds, mint, and cilantro and gently toss to combine. Sprinkle with salt and pepper to taste. Serve.

Chickpea-Spinach Bulgur

Prep Time: 5 min

Cook Time: 20 min

Serve: 6

Ingredients:

- ¾ cup chicken or vegetable broth
- ¾ cup water
- 1 (15-oz.) can chickpeas, rinsed
- 1 cup medium-grind bulgur, rinsed
- 1 onion, chopped fine
- 1 tbsp. lemon juice
- 2 tbsp. za'atar
- 3 garlic cloves, minced
- 3 oz. (3 cups) baby spinach, chopped
- 3 tbsp. extra-virgin olive oil
- Salt and pepper

Preparation:

1. Heat 2 tbsp. oil in a big saucepan on moderate heat until it starts to shimmer. Put in onion and ½ tsp. salt and cook till they become tender, approximately five minutes. Mix in garlic and 1 tbsp. za'atar and cook until aromatic, approximately half a minute.

2. Mix in bulgur, chickpeas, broth, and water and bring to simmer. Decrease heat to low, cover, and simmer gently until bulgur is tender, 16 to 18 minutes.

3. Remove from the heat, lay clean dish towel underneath lid and let bulgur sit for about ten minutes. Put in spinach, lemon juice, remaining 1 tbsp. za'atar, and residual 1 tbsp. oil and fluff gently with fork to combine. Sprinkle with salt and pepper to taste. Serve.

Classic Baked Brown Rice

Prep Time: 10 min

Cook Time: 20 min

Serve: 6

Ingredients:

- 1½ cups long-grain brown rice, rinsed
- 2 tsp. extra-virgin olive oil
- 2 1/3 cups boiling water
- Salt and pepper

Preparation:

1. Place the oven rack in the centre of the oven and pre-heat your oven to 375°F. Mix boiling water, rice, oil, and ½ tsp. salt in 8-inch square baking dish. Cover dish tightly using double layer of aluminium foil. Bake until rice becomes soft and water is absorbed, about 1 hour.

Remove the dish from oven, uncover, and gently fluff rice with fork, scraping up any rice stuck to the bottom.

2. Cover dish with clean dish towel and let rice sit for about five minutes. Uncover and let rice sit for about five minutes longer. Sprinkle with salt and pepper to taste. Serve.

Classic Italian Seafood Risotto

Prep Time: 10 min

Cook Time: 20 min

Serve: 4

Ingredients:

- 1/8 tsp. saffron threads, crumbled
- 1 (14.5-oz.) can diced tomatoes, drained
- 1 cup dry white wine
- 1 onion, chopped fine
- 1 tbsp. lemon juice
- 1 tsp. minced fresh thyme or ¼ tsp. dried
- 12 oz. large shrimp (26 to 30 per lb.), peeled and deveined, shells reserved
- 12 oz. small bay scallops
- 2 bay leaves
- 2 cups Arborio rice

- 2 cups chicken broth
- 2 tbsp. minced fresh parsley
- 2½ cups water
- 4 (8-oz.) bottles clam juice
- 5 garlic cloves, minced
- 5 tbsp. extra-virgin olive oil
- Salt and pepper

Preparation:

1. Bring shrimp shells, broth, water, clam juice, tomatoes, and bay leaves to boil in a big saucepan on moderate to high heat. Decrease the heat to a simmer and cook for 20 minutes. Strain mixture through fine-mesh strainer into big container, pressing on solids to extract as much liquid as possible; discard solids. Return broth to now-empty saucepan, cover, and keep warm on low heat.

2. Heat 2 tbsp. oil in a Dutch oven on moderate heat until it starts to shimmer. Put in onion and cook till they become tender, approximately five minutes.

3. Put in rice, garlic, thyme, and saffron and cook, stirring often, until grain edges begin to turn translucent, approximately three minutes.

4. Put in wine and cook, stirring often, until fully absorbed, approximately three minutes. Mix in 3½ cups warm broth, bring to simmer, and cook, stirring

intermittently, until almost fully absorbed, about fifteen minutes.

5. Carry on cooking rice, stirring often and adding warm broth, 1 cup at a time, every few minutes as liquid is absorbed, until rice is creamy and cooked through but still somewhat firm in center, about fifteen minutes.

6. Mix in shrimp and scallops and cook, stirring often, until opaque throughout, approximately three minutes. Remove pot from heat, cover, and allow to sit for about five minutes.

7. Adjust consistency with remaining warm broth as required (you may have broth left over). Mix in remaining 3 tbsp. oil, parsley, and lemon juice and sprinkle with salt and pepper to taste. Serve.

Classic Stovetop White Rice

Prep Time: 10 min

Cook Time: 10 min

Serve: 6

Ingredients:

- 1 tbsp. extra-virgin olive oil
- 2 cups long-grain white rice, rinsed
- 3 cups water
- long-grain rice can substitute basmati, jasmine, or Texmati rice for the long-grain rice.
- Salt and pepper

Preparation:

1. Heat oil in a big saucepan on moderate heat until it starts to shimmer. Put in rice and cook, stirring frequently, until grain edges begin to turn translucent, approximately two minutes. Put in water and 1 tsp. salt and bring to simmer.

2. Cover, decrease the heat to low, and simmer gently until rice becomes soft and water is absorbed, approximately twenty minutes. Remove from the heat, lay clean dish towel underneath lid and let rice sit for about ten minutes.

3. Gently fluff rice with fork. Sprinkle with salt and pepper to taste. Serve.

Chicken Sausage Minestrone

Ingredients:

- 4 sliced chicken sausage
- 4 tomatoes; sliced and peeled
- 2 chopped cloves
- ½ pound of diced green beans
- 2 sliced carrots
- A dubbed zucchini
- Olive oil;
- 2 tablespoons
- 1 diced sweet onion
- ½ cup of green peas; frozen
- 1 sliced celery stalk
- 2 cups of vegetable stalk
- ½ cup of marjoram; dried
- Water; 6 cups

- ½ teaspoon of oregano; dried
- ½ teaspoon of basil; dried
- Pepper and salt to taste

Preparation:

1. Get a soup pot and heat the oil, then pour in your chicken sausage and some diced onion, then cook for 5 minutes.

2. Now, add in your tomatoes, carrot, cloves, onion and celery and wait till it's cooked for another 10 minutes then add your remaining Ingredients. Add pepper and salt to taste, then cook for 20 minutes.

3. Serve and enjoy your soup when warm.

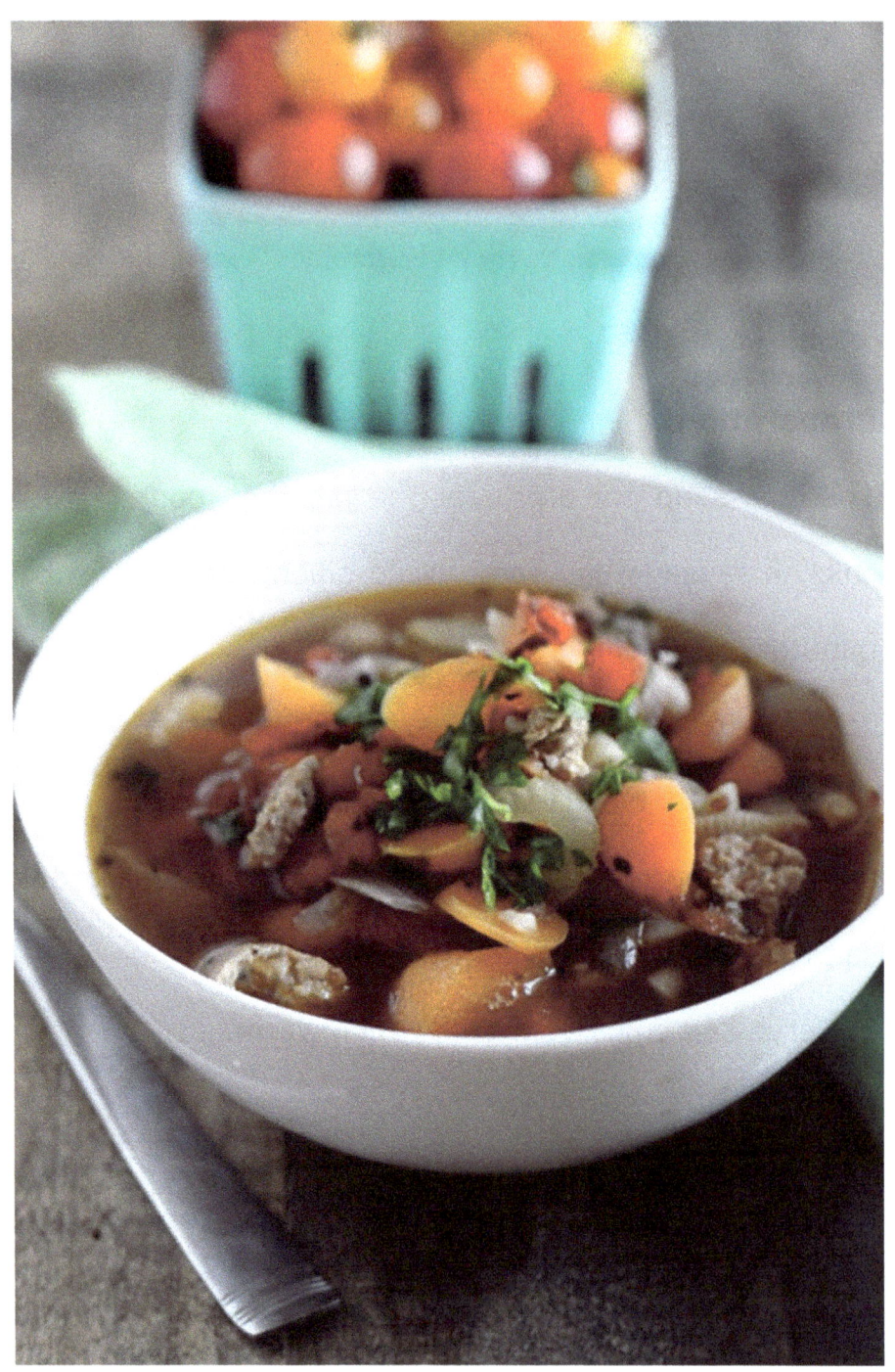

Italian Lentil soup

Ingredients:

- 2 tablespoons of sliced parsley
- Tomato paste; 2 tablespoons
- Olive Oil; 2 tablespoons
- 2 sliced cloves
- 1 cup of sliced tomatoes
- 2 celery stalks; chopped
- 2 sliced shallots
- 2 carrots; chopped
- ¼ cup of red wine
- Water; 6 cups
- A basil sprig
- A thyme sprigs
- An oregano sprig
- Green lentils; 1 cup

- 2 cups of vegetable stock
- Pepper and salt to taste
-

Preparation:

1. Get a soup pot and heat your olive oil, then pour in your chopped celery, clove, carrots and shallot, then cook for 5 minutes before adding your vegetable stock, lentils, tomatoes, wine and water.

2. Join in the herbs, then add pepper and salt to taste and then cook for 25 minutes.

3. After 25 minutes, add your sliced parsley in and serve your warm soup.

Smoked chicken sausage soup

Ingredients:

- 2 sliced chicken sausage
- 2 sliced smoked chicken sausage
- 1 can of sliced tomatoes
- 1 onion, sliced
- Water; 2 cups
- Vegetable stock; 2 cups
- 1 celery stalk; chopped
- Chopped cilantro; 2 tablespoons
- Olive Oil; 2 tablespoons
- Pepper and salt to taste

Preparation:

1. Get a soup pot and heat your olive oil, then pour in your sausage and cook for 5 minutes. After that, pour in your sliced onion, tomatoes, celery and carrots and cook for another 5 minutes.

2. Now, add your short pasta and water with pepper and salt to taste, then cook for 20 minutes. After 20 minutes, pour in your chopped parsley and cilantro then serve after cooling.

Bulgur, Kale and Cheese Mix

Prep Time: 10 min

Cook Time: 10 min

Serve: 6

Ingredients:

- 4 ounces bulgur
- 4 ounces kale, chopped
- 1 tablespoon mint, chopped
- 3 spring onions, chopped
- 1 cucumber, chopped
- A pinch of allspice, ground
- 2 tablespoons olive oil
- Zest and juice of ½ lemon
- 4 ounces feta cheese, crumbled

Preparation:

1. Put bulgur in a bowl, cover with hot water, aside for 10 minutes and fluff with a fork.

2. Heat a pan with the oil over medium heat, add the onions and the allspice and cook for 3 minutes. Add the bulgur and the rest of the ingredients, cook everything for 5-6 minutes more, divide between plates and serve.

Lemon Chicken Soup

Prep Time: 10 min

Cook Time: 20 min

Serve: 6

Ingredients:

- 10 cups chicken broth
- 3 tbsp. olive oil
- 8 cloves garlic, minced
- 1 sweet onion, sliced
- 1 large lemon, zested
- 2 boneless skinless chicken breasts
- 1 cup Israeli couscous
- 1/2 tsp. crushed red pepper
- 2 oz. crumbled feta
- 1/3 cup chopped chive
- Salt and pepper, to taste

Preparation:

1. Grab a stock pot, add the oil and place over a medium heat. Add the onion and garlic and cook for five minutes until soft. Add the broth, chicken breasts, lemon zest and crushed pepper.

2. Raise the heat, cover and bring to a boil. Reduce the heat then simmer for 5 minutes. Turn off the heat, remove the lid and remove the chicken from the pot.

3. Pop onto a place and use two forks to shred. Pop back into the pot, add the feta, chives and salt and pepper.

4. Stir well then serve and enjoy.

Tuscan Vegetable Pasta Soup

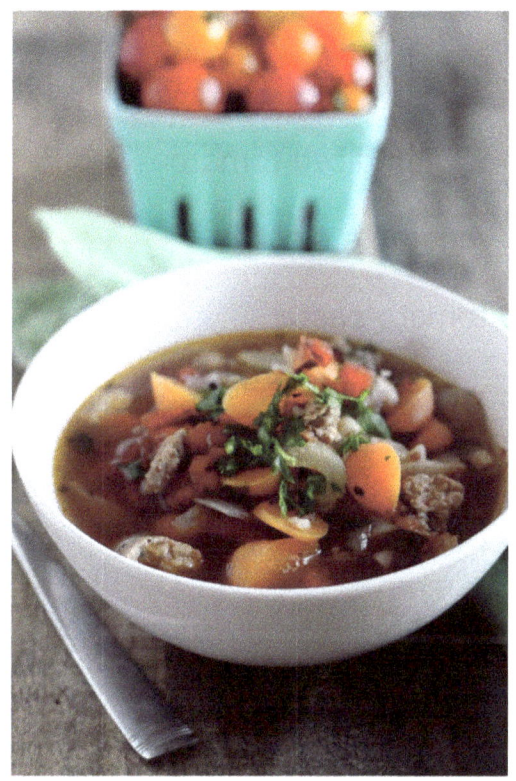

Prep Time: 10 min

Cook Time: 30 min

Serve: 6

Ingredients:

- 2 tbsp. extra virgin olive oil

- 4 cloves garlic, minced
- 1 medium yellow onion, diced
- 1/2 cup carrot, chopped
- 1/2 cup celery, chopped
- 1 medium zucchini, sliced and quartered
- 1 x 15 oz. can diced tomatoes
- 6 cups vegetable stock
- 2 tbsp. tomato paste
- 6-8 oz. whole wheat pasta
- 1 x 15 oz. can white beans
- 2 large handfuls baby spinach
- 6 basil cubes
- Salt and pepper, to taste
- Fresh chopped parsley, for garnish

Preparation:

1. Grab a stock pot, add the oil and pop over a medium heat.

2. Add the onion and garlic and cook for five minutes until soft. Throw in the carrots, celery and zucchini and cook for an extra 5 minutes, stirring occasionally.

3. Add the tomato and salt and pepper and cook for 1-2 minutes. Add the veggies broth and tomato paste, stir well then bring to the boil. Throw in the pasta, cook for 10 minutes then add the spinach, white beans, basil cubes and seasoning. Stir well then remove from the heat.

4. Divide between large bowls and serve and enjoy.

Dairy Free Zucchini Soup

Prep Time: 10 min

Cook Time: 25 min

Serve: 8

Ingredients:

- 2½ lb. zucchini
- 1 medium onion, diced
- 2 tbsp. olive oil
- 4 garlic cloves, chopped
- 4 cups chicken stock
- Sea salt and pepper, to taste
- 1/3 cup fresh basil leaves

Preparation:

1. Grab a pan, add the oil and pop over a medium heat. Add the onion, garlic and zucchini and cook for five minutes until soft. Add the stock and simmer for 15 minutes.

2. Remove from the heat, stir through the basil, add the seasoning and use an immersion blender to whizz until smooth. Serve and enjoy.

Farro Stew with Kale & Cannellini Beans

Prep Time: 10 min

Cook Time: 1 h

Serve: 4

Ingredients:

- 2 tbsp. olive oil
- 2 medium carrots, diced
- 1 medium onion, chopped
- 2 sticks celery, chopped
- 4 cloves garlic, minced
- 5 cups low-sodium vegetable broth
- 1 x 14.5 oz. can diced tomatoes
- 1 cup farro, rinsed
- 1 tsp. dried oregano
- 1 bay leaf
- Salt, to taste

- 1/2 cup parsley
- 4 cups chopped kale, thick ribs removed
- 1 x 15 oz. can cannellini beans, drained and rinsed
- 1 tbsp. fresh lemon juice
- 1/2 cup feta cheese, crumbled

Preparation:

1. Grab a stock pot, add the oil and place over a medium heat. Add the onion, carrots and celery and cook for five minutes until becoming soft.

2. Add the garlic and cook for another 30 seconds. Stir through the broth, tomatoes, farro, oregano, bay leaf, parsley and salt.

3. Cover with the lid and bring to the boil. Reduce the heat then simmer for 20 minutes. Remove the lid, add the kale and cook for a further 10-15 minutes.

4. Remove the bay leaf, add the beans, stir through the lemon juice and any additional liquid then stir well to combine. Serve and enjoy.

Italian Meatball Soup

Prep Time: 10 min

Cook Time: 45 min

Serve: 6

Ingredients:

- 1/4 - 1/2 cup freshly grated parmesan cheese (optional)
- 1 free-range egg
- 1 cup breadcrumbs, optional
- 2 tbsp. fresh parsley, minced
- 1 tsp. dried oregano
- 1/2 tsp. sea salt
- ½ tsp. black pepper
- 3 tbsp. olive oil
- 2 quarts chicken broth or beef broth
- 3 tbsp. tomato paste

- 1 onion, diced
- 2 bay leaves
- 4-5 sprigs fresh thyme
- ½ tsp. whole black peppercorns
- Fresh parmesan cheese, grated
- 1-2 tbsp. fresh basil leaves, torn 1-2 tbsp. fresh parsley, chopped
- Salt and pepper, to taste

Preparation:

1. Place all the meatball ingredients except the oil into a medium bowl. Using your hands, mix well and form into meatballs. Place the oil into a stock pot, place over a medium heat and add the meatballs, browning on all sides.

2. Remove the meatballs from the pan. Add more oil to the pan if needed and then add the onion. Cook for five minutes until soft. Add the remaining soup ingredients, stir well then cook for 10 minutes.

3. Return the meatballs to the pan and simmer for a few minutes to warm through. Serve and enjoy.

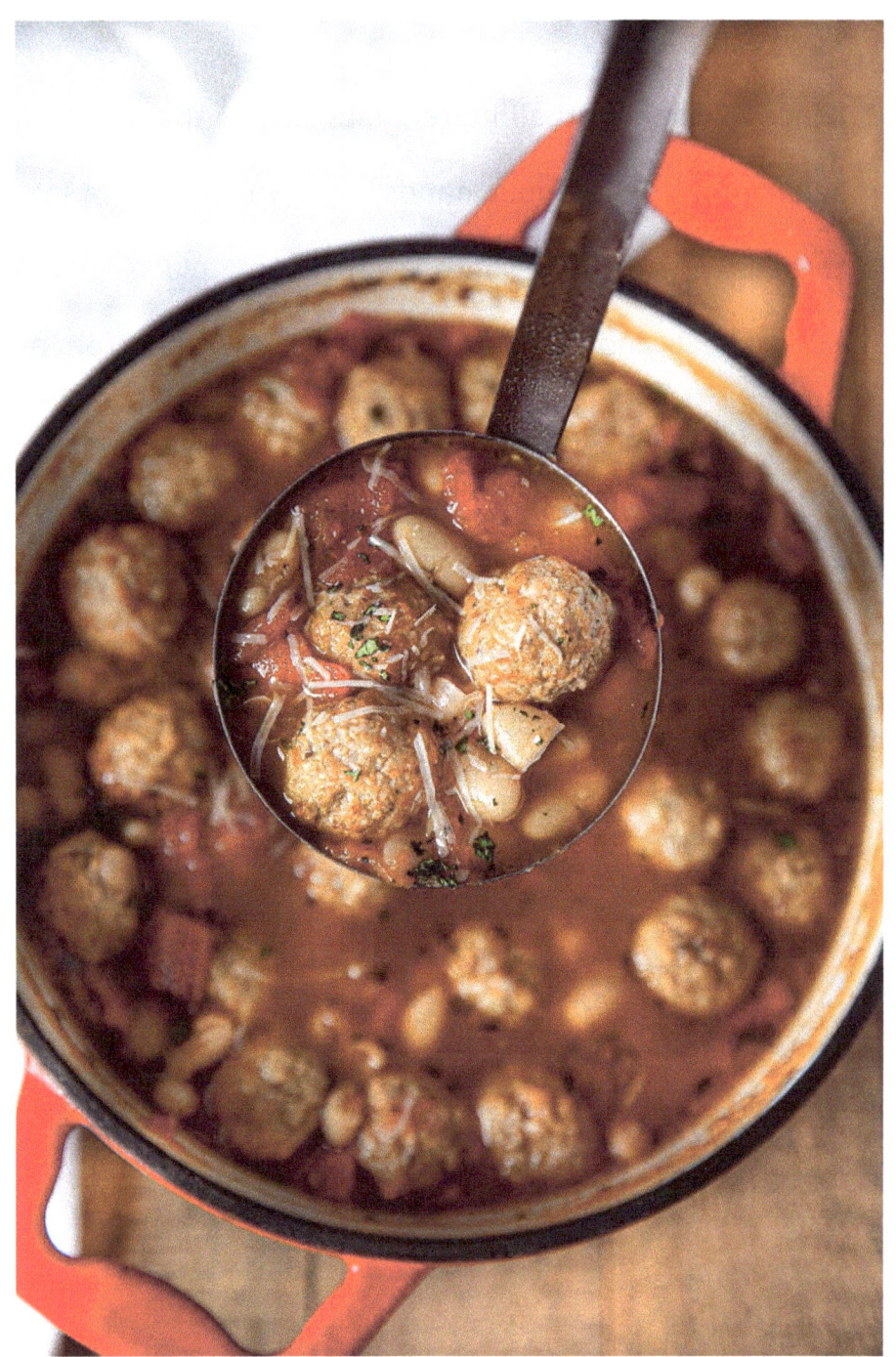

www.ingramcontent.com/pod-product-compliance
Lightning Source LLC
Chambersburg PA
CBHW070730030426
42336CB00013B/1936